Why Not Me?

Also by Linda Ray McBride
Mema Has Cancer

Why Not Me?

LINDA MCBRIDE

inspiring Voices®
A Service of Guideposts

Inspiring Voices books may be ordered through booksellers or by contacting:

Inspiring Voices
1663 Liberty Drive
Bloomington, IN 47403
www.inspiringvoices.com
1-(866) 697-5313

Because of the dynamic nature of the Internet, any web addresses or links contained in this book may have changed since publication and may no longer be valid. The views expressed in this work are solely those of the author and do not necessarily reflect the views of the publisher, and the publisher hereby disclaims any responsibility for them.

Certain stock imagery © Thinkstock.
Any people depicted in stock imagery provided by Thinkstock are models, and such images are being used for illustrative purposes only.

ISBN: 978-1-4624-0209-0 (e)
ISBN: 978-1-4624-0208-3 (sc)

Library of Congress Control Number: 2012942543

Printed in the United States of America

Inspiring Voices rev. date: 8/01/2012

Preface

I doubted everything. What was wrong? I was spiritual but so afraid; I loved my life and feared the suffering. I had to prepare myself and my family for a time that would change our lives forever.

Dear God give me the strength to survive.

Acknowledgement

Mcdonald Baptist Church I will always be thankful for your prayers, endless meals, just right amount of visits, calls and the fact that you were available for my family and understood when I was too sick for visits. Also my wonderful husband, children, grand kids who kept me full of hope when I wanted to give up. Bob, you are the love of my life. Hunter, Hannah, Micah, Sarah, Cade and Braylon, you are the sweetest grand kids, full of love, joy, and always surprises. Tommy, Amanda and David, you are the strength that makes a mother so proud and thankful every day for having children.

Introduction

We can feel discouraged, disappointed and selfish longing for life as it was, and then we see another person that is much worse. Realizing I have no right to question, why this happened to us. I will continue to pray and believe

I will survive.

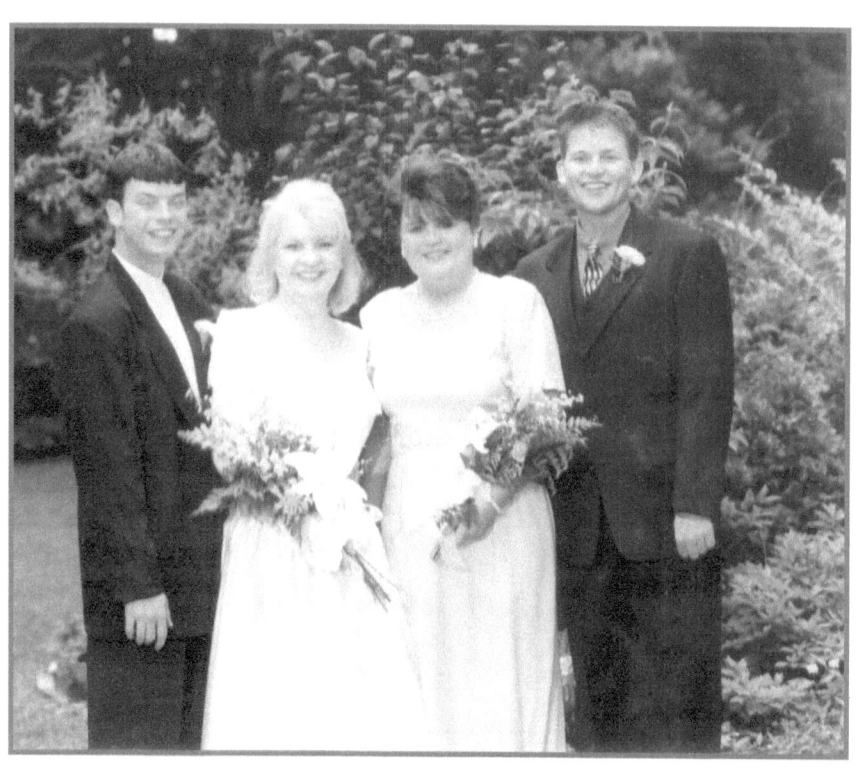

Cancer can never extinguish Love

———— ✿ ————

Chapter 1

The Diagnosis

I looked over at my daughter and was happy she was with me. I was so blessed to have my children so close. I had gone to the emergency room with a drug reaction to the antibiotic Doctor Lee had prescribed after the neck biopsy. Just 6 months earlier we had the big cancer scare, a spot on my lung had enlarged and the Doctor was convinced it was cancer and needed to be removed quickly. The surgery was very intensive and a long painful recovery. The spot was benign and I was a lucky patient the Doctor said. I knew I was blessed and was so thankful to everyone and felt very close to God through all of the recovery. The day before I went in for the surgery a lump appeared on the right side of my neck. Doctor Heida said we would just watch it and if it was there in two weeks to see my primary care giver. Now I was under the care of Doctor Lee who was watching my neck and felt it was nothing because the size did get smaller in a month, but never went away. He reassured me it would be fine. I was having headaches and night sweats. The Doctor thought this was hormonal and prescribed a larger dose of compound hormone therapy. I remember one night waking up from a dream, wet with perspiration and head pounding. I told Bob, my very concerned husband, that I felt my body was fighting very hard to get well. Something was not right I had been very healthy before the lung surgery. He told me to call the Doctor and let him check me out. Doctor Lee reassured me that if I was his wife he would just continue to watch the lump and he did order a sleep study. Thinking this may explain the headaches in the mornings. The sleep study was essentially normal but he decided to repair a deviated septum to help me breath better and relieve the morning headaches. I went in for the pre-op exam and the lymph node in my neck was enlarged more and he said while he had me asleep for the nose he would remove the lymph node. I would not have to worry about it anymore. I had the surgery and he knew it was bad right away, but waited on the pathology report before telling me. I had a rough day the day I went home after surgery. I was laying back in Bob's recliner with an ice pack on my neck. I was feeling a deep down nausea that erupted like a violent volcano. Tommy put a fresh glass of water on the table and a new Ice pack on my neck. I looked in his eyes and saw all his concern as he wiped a tear from my cheek. He said, "Oh my God there is blood in your tears." That night a poem came in my head and I got up and wrote it quickly, before I forgot that moment we had shared.

Blood Stained Tears

My firstborn looked so compassionately in my eyes, as a tear fell going toward my ear. He wiped it gently and said Oh my God there is blood in your tears. I told him it was probably normal after the nose job, I had feared.

I had my nose fixed so I would no longer snore or maybe, I should say roar.

I reassured him as I saw his deep concern and loving compassion. I told him he always got bewildered when things go the least bit wrong. When he saw blood it was hard to be strong.

When he was 10 his sister fell and cut her arm I told him to bring me a towel as I looked at her arm and tried to calm everyone down. After seeing the blood on her arm he ran in every room and shouted I can't find a towel. He opened the refrigerator as if the towel would be there. Panic in his voice he shouted again I could not find one. I told him to look in the bathroom. David, his younger brother had already brought me a towel. He was calm and had taken care of the problem as a younger brother would. Tommy had that same panic look as he wiped my tear, but he did not run. I patted his hand and said Lord please help Tommy be strong. This is just the beginning of our blood stained tears and God we will need you to stay near. Doctor Lee did tell Bob it was cancer. I had done all the right things. I did not smoke or drink gotten all my well checkups, very health conscious. I had never lived with a smoker. Now I was waiting in the hospital for this visit from Doctor Lee to tell me the results. It was a beautiful day in November 2006. Doctor Lee entered the room he was neat and wearing a tie on Saturday. He looked so young, tall and slim. But today he had old eyes, he looked at me and I sat up smiled big, I was ready to go home feeling better. I was anxious to see my grandchildren, and let them see I was fine. Bob walked over to my bed and stood close to me and put his hand on my back. Doctor Lee looked at Amanda, my sweet usually very emotional daughter, and said. You don't know how hard my walk from my office was this morning. He looked at me and Amanda walked to the other side of my bed. He said you have cancer. I felt my tears filling my eyes as my voice trembled. I felt a tear fall on my arm it was Bob's. Amanda said very calmly, what do we need to do first and we will do it and get through this and Mama you will be O.K. I looked at Bob, he had been my rock and I felt the love I had for this man and how hard this was on him and my children. I had to think and plan, I could only think of one thing, I have cancer. I could die. I felt so safe and close to Bob. I hurt for him, how do we prepare the kids and the grandkids for what is ahead. We both had been married before and really appreciated our loving relationship so much. The holidays were just ahead and we enjoyed them so much with our kids and grandkids. Now how do I plan any celebration? I have to prepare for more surgery and treatment. Wiping my eyes and trying to speak, I asked Doctor Lee, what do I do next? He said I am referring you to Doctor Christine, she is a Surgeon at the Medical College of Georgia and very good. She is out of town until after the Thanksgiving Holidays and you need time to heal from this surgery. You will see her as soon as possible and have more surgery, chemo and radiation. This is a tough treatment and you will need a lot of follow up. We don't know where the primary cancer is. I felt my body trembling and Bob had his hand on my back. I felt so heavy I could not imagine this, I just had a PET Scan and it was normal. I had major surgery on my lung five months ago and it was benign. We have to do aggressive treatment. I nodded and Bob said we would do whatever we have to do, to get her well. He said come back into my office on Monday. The nurse came in and told Bob to drive to the front and she would take me down. Bob left I went to the Bathroom and prayed. God please help me know what to do what to say and to remember you are in control. I got in the wheel chair and tried to hold my head up. I told the nurse I am ready. She said I hope you feel better soon and have a good holiday. I said they just told me I have cancer. She put her arm around me and said I will pray for you. The Tears fell again she said that is OK just let it out. The elevator door closed and I took a deep breath; I had not even been breathing regular. I had worked at the hospital and I knew the routine, but this time it was so foreign. I tried to speak again but no sound came out of my mouth.

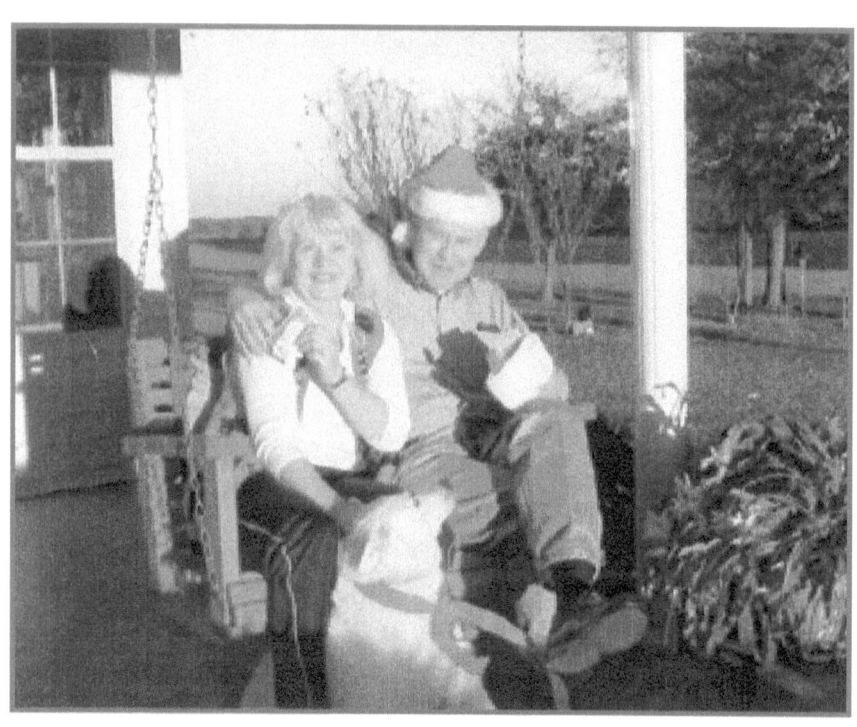

I Love Christmas

Chapter 2

Why?

Tears came again. Amanda had gone to pick up the children and meet us at home. She had been calm and reassuring. I remember now the Doctor had said I was healthy and not underweight and no family history of cancer and had excellent family support. This was all good. I remembered all he had said and kept hearing it in my head. The nurse said we are at the pick-up area and your husband will bring the car. The tears fell again and she said remember God will help you, I said thank you but it was just a whisper. I had always prayed and had a great faith, but God Why??Why??Why?? Bob pulled up and got out to help me get in the car. He asked do you want to get something to eat. I said I just want to go home. I wanted to talk to the children. I needed to call Mama. I wanted things to be normal, but things were not normal. I had to fight hard for my life, and it had just begun. Because of the holidays it was hard to schedule appointments and make plans. My sons Tommy and David were so stressed. Tommy had personal challenges and I knew this news would make him so restless and wondered what he would do. He would not always take his medicine and take care of himself. I pray daily for him. He is so unpredictable and history has proven that he has made a lot of bad choices. The only other time I had felt so afraid was when Tommy told me he had a severe medical condition. David on the other coast was on the Internet researching neck cancer treatments and outcomes. He emailed my Doctor and she emailed him back. We did have a wonderful informative Doctor. I prayed but I still wondered WHY? WHY? More Surgery On December 8, 2006 I had a neck resection, this was very extensive and they removed my vein, tonsil areas and lymph nodes also the neck muscle. I was not prepared for this. My doctor had prepared my son and he had viewed a lot of cases on the Internet but advised me not to look and just trust my Doctor and I did. Doctor Christine was wonderful and had a great team. I became the patient and totally trusted their care. After a week I was home and had someone with me around the clock. The pain was severe but I did get relief from medication that had a very bad effect on my gut. Christmas came and went I was unable to do all the things we normally did. David decorated and we had a lot of good food, but I could hardly eat. I just planned to make up for this holiday next Christmas. I would really celebrate Christmas 2007. I was physically unable to do anything for over 10 minutes.

Chapter 3

Plan of Care

The plan was to see the radiation Doctor and Chemo Doctor in January as soon as possible. Again we had to wait because of all the holidays. My first visit was for the plan of care by radiation. Doctor Weems said we need to get you a feeding tube. He stated I would not be able to eat after the radiation started and wanted the tube in before. I could not believe this, I had not thought about that, but I was losing weight and still eating all I could and drinking the enriched milk shakes. He also wanted me to see my Dentist and have a mold made to protect my teeth during radiation and get fluoride treatment. I had to update my day planner; I had so many appointments and follow up with all my physicians. The next week I saw the surgeon to get the tube and also the Chemo Oncologist, Doctor Robertson and he was so kind and compassionate I knew he would be wonderful also. The plan was 6 chemo treatments once a week and 35 radiations 5 times a week. I can't tell you how afraid I was. The weakness, nausea, and tiredness were overwhelming. I had never been so tired I could not get up and now it was such an effort to even roll over in bed. I wanted to talk to the children more but did not have the energy. Dear God I am afraid for my kids. I read healing scriptures listened to tapes and prayed. Dear God please give me the Strength to Survive. Finally the Chemo and Radiation was over. It was the middle of March and in February I had to be admitted to the hospital for severe dehydration and ulcers in my mouth. That was quiet an ordeal nothing seem to stop the vomiting. The Chemo had poisoned my system so badly; I had to stop treatment for 10 days. I begged the Doctor to give me a break and he did but increased the Chemo for another week. I had 7 chemo treatments and was so happy when the last radiation and chemo was over. I now had a suction machine by my bed that did help when the mucus became so thick I felt I would choke. I begged God to help me, and I only needed the machine a couple of months. The nurses at the radiation center gave me a beautiful plant with pink blooms. I was so relieved but threw up all the way home. My sister in law had driven me to radiation after the kids had to go back to work and Bob was working also. I told her she was heaven sent and she was. I left a lot of DNA in her car and we just kept towels, pans, and Phenergan in the car and she would stop and assist me when I could only lean over and vomit over and over. That day I knew would not last forever. We stopped and I opened the car door, but could not stand up. She came and helped me into the house. I opened my bedroom door and what a Surprise you could not see anything but beautiful balloons and flowers with a sign that said. Congratulations you have finished treatments. We Love you So Much, Tommy, Amanda & David. A book was on my bed that said "Why Daughters need Mothers. A guardian angel music box played you are the wind beneath my wings. I wanted to call all of them and say thank you, everything is so beautiful and all my favorite colors. But the nausea started again and Ann helped me in bed and gave me more Phenergan on my wrist and it was a wonderful drug it helped so much. After the nausea stopped, she gave me pain medicine and soon I was sleeping.

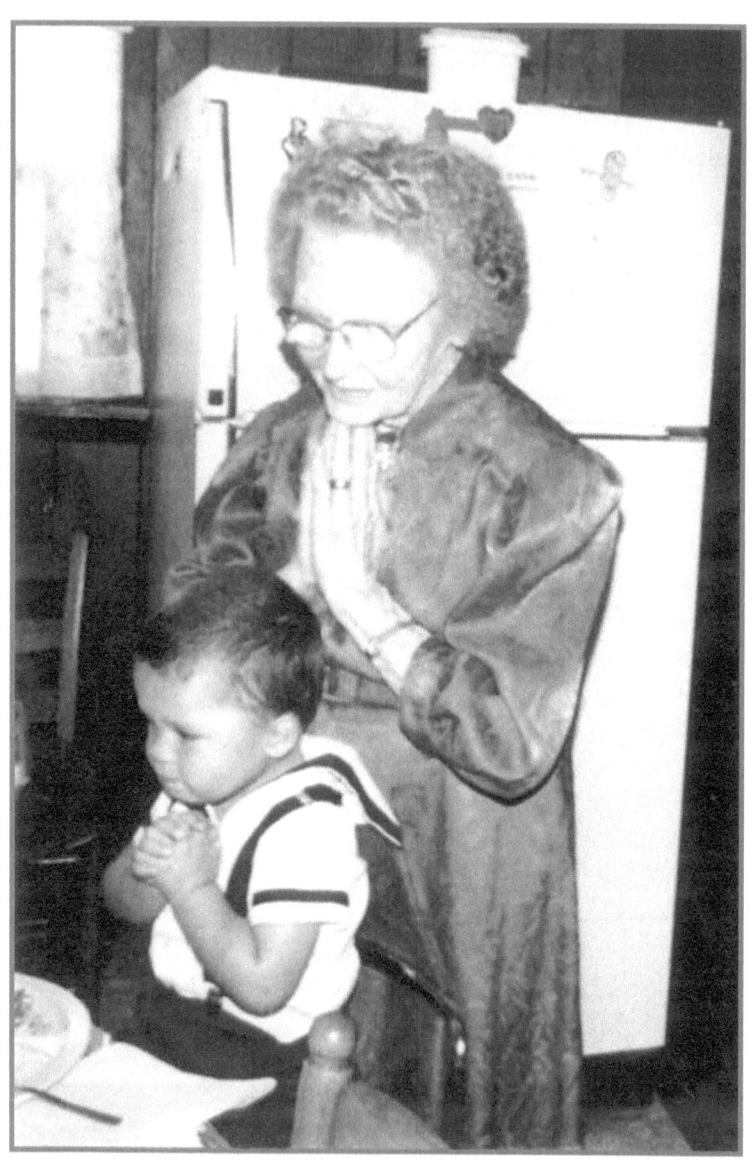

A Mother's Prayer

Chapter 4

───────── ✿ ─────────

The Dream

I was dreaming about eating and all the kids and grandkids were around the table and Bob prayed and thanked God I was healed. That dream gave me so much comfort that when I woke up. I called the kids and they all said you sound so much better. Things would get better now. I still pray daily for advanced drug therapy that will help cancer patients with pain and nausea. The side effects of chemo are so hard but radiation was even worse. Chemo you would have a few days between treatments that the nausea would stop. But, radiation was every day and you were sick every day. My mouth tongue and lips were sore, raw and had sores in and out of my mouth. Who was the woman in the mirror? My hair fell out on the right side of my head and back of my head that was the least thing I worried about. I had thick blond hair and unless you looked close you could not tell. I just brushed it back and down over to the right side. The last visit for radiation, I saw others that were just starting they looked so different than me. I had red swollen neck and face. I had lost 36 pounds and had not felt like shopping my clothes were too big, Ann had gotten me some things and Amanda had shopped for me some. I just did not want a lot of small things because I knew I would gain some weight soon. I had a lot of new clothes from Christmas I had not even worn. Now, even my shoes were too big. I wondered how in the world that could happen. So Ann stopped and picked me up some shoes a size smaller. All of that was hard but the thing that was so hard was the fact I could not brush my teeth without so much pain. It was so hard to swallow I was glad I had the feeding tube. Bob had become so good at putting food and medicine in the tube. I ate Yogurt daily and hoped it would help the soreness and keep the swallowing active. I would do this while the pain medicine was working at its peak. I would then lie very still and cover my head and pray. God please help me. I tried hard not to complain, my family was so worried and Bob was not resting at night and still trying to work all the days possible. My brother, Steve, had had surgery and was now on a ventilator. My poor mother had two very sick children and I prayed so hard for Steve and her. I knew they were trying to keep any bad news away from me and my white count was so low that I could not visit the hospital and we had to be careful about exposure to any colds or sickness. My mother was 86 and very frail and I cried for her. Mama would tell me God is in control I do not understand all this but we will get through it and be stronger. Her faith was so strong even when I was so low. My oldest brother, Larry, was a minister and he helped Mom and visited Steve and me often. I told him please stay healthy and he smiled big and said I will.

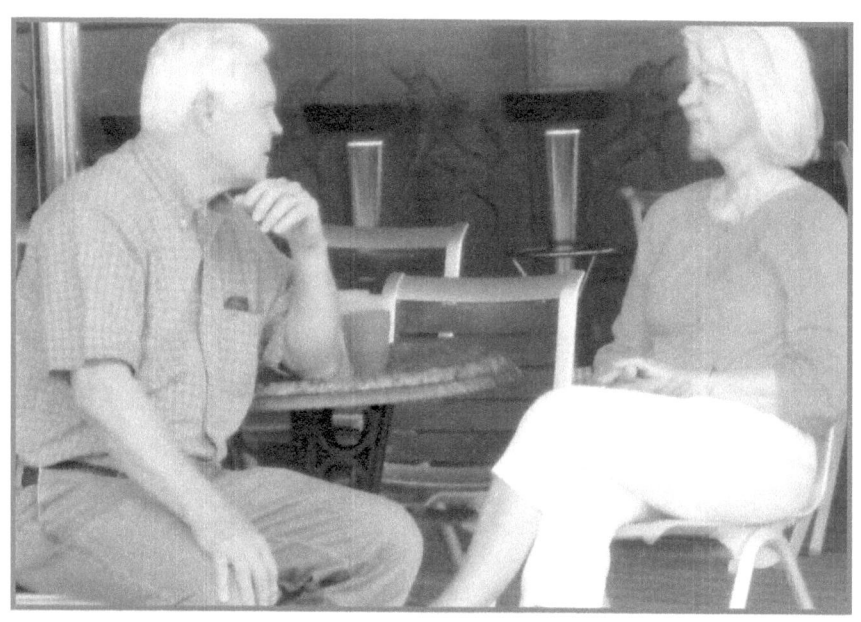

Decisions

Chapter 5

Side Effects

Three months passed and I had a very sore and stiff neck. I knew I was getting better and I was going to physical therapy three to four times a week and the therapist was very pleased with my progress. Now I started having a very high blood pressure and Doctor Geraldo changed my medicine. I started taking Norvace and after three days my feet were swelling and I had no energy. I would shampoo my hair and would have to rest before I could blow-dry it. Every simple task was so hard. I would keep thinking the cancer is coming back and then I would pray and ask God help me have the faith to say I know I am healed and I can be encouraging to others going through this ordeal. The cancer is so horrible and robs you of the feeling that everything is OK. I decided that I would try to go into the office and do some light work. I missed everyone and especially the residents. I still was not ready to drive, my friend, KaSandra said she would pick me up and take me home whenever I was ready. She was a blessing and had always encouraged me. She never hesitated to help me no matter what I tried to do. I opened the car door and KaSandra said, "God is so Good." And she had such a beautiful smile that I felt much better. I would force myself to go to work most days, I had to stay in the office more than I wanted, but I did not have enough energy to walk the halls and visit. I loved talking and spending time with the residents. They had wonderful stories. Each one had a special place in my heart and they always told me, "not to overdo it." "We will come to your office or send for you if we need to." They were trying to take care of me. I knew the ones that would come by the office, but 35% of the resident could not visit or express their needs. I could tell when they were stressed by their eyes. It takes a while but you learn all the signs of pain, fear, discomfort, and anxiety in each one. When you see a smile from a resident that has been very depressed it is wonderful. Reaching out to touch the hand and talk for a while does wonders, for you and the resident. When my mother in law was deep into the disease of Alzheimer's she would have moments that she thought she was still at home and taking care of her 12 children. I asked her one day. "How was your day?" She said, "I am so tired, I worked all day." Then she said" go and eat, I fixed a big supper, it is on the table." Smiling she said, "I am going to rest now." I would never tell her she was in the nursing home and she was in the wheelchair and had to be lifted and put to bed to rest. She just closed her eyes to rest and had a wonderful expression on her face. No, her reality was much worse, she had to receive total care, and she could no longer walk, go to the bathroom and remember to eat. Our next visit Bob asked, Mama why did you whip me so much? She said I did not do it half enough. We all laughed she was having a good day. She had that sparkle in her eye and a mischievous look. She lived in a different time in her mind and that was good, because the reality was hard. Her world was a small room in the nursing home and the memories that kept her content. She had a stroke a few weeks later and the Doctor said we would just keep her comfortable. All the kids visited often and the day she died Ann and I were in the room to see the beautiful expression on her face when in the twinkling of an eye she went to heaven. We knew we had witnessed a beautiful thing when she opened her eyes with the expression of a child on Christmas Morning. She had a beautiful glow and we approached each side of her bed. Ann said, "Mama," as she closed her eyes and the life left her and we had such a peace and presence in the room. We felt as if we had received a wonderful gift. We saw an expression of someone looking into heaven. I had been in health care for 30 years and that is a moment I will always cherish and never forget. Maybe she was helping me not to fear death, not knowing the future and I would be fighting for my life. Now it was getting warm and the May weather was wonderful. I had a follow up visit with Doctor Christine and she was pleased with my improvement and how my surgery had healed. The Speech therapist stated I needed more bio feedback therapy. She was a walking doll and had a personality of an angel. I wanted to do all she requested because she had encouraged me so much. She even said I would be able to sing in the choir again. I did not know how, my voice was so harsh and cracked so much, no one recognized me on the phone any more. When I would say this is Linda they would pause and say you sound so different I thought it was Bob. My cousin called and I had always nagged him for smoking we had a special bond and he knew I was so down. He said God you sound sexy like an old smoker. I said you know the only smoke I get is from talking on the phone with you. We laughed and he said hell this is not fair I smoke like a freight train and you get cancer. I agreed and added when are you going to stop and he said when I couldn't get to a cigarette. We had always teased and shared good times and bad times. I knew he would do anything to make me feel better. He told me a joke and laughed with such energy I smiled and laughed at him. He said hang on girl I will see you soon. I was disappointed I had to take more therapy; I was tired and wanted to return to work. I wanted to try to get back my energy I missed everyone at the nursing home and I knew it would cheer me up just being with the residents and the staff. I received a card from Janice, my dear friend of 25 years, "Refuse to be discouraged when the storm clouds come your way, but trust that in tomorrow you will find a brighter day. Refuse to be discouraged when you're faced with doubts and fears, but keep on pressing onward for the joy beyond tears. Refuse to be discouraged, and in time you will understand that courage comes by simple faith in God's sweet guiding hand." And her inside note said, "Linda may God strengthen with patience as you wait for trials to cease; may He fill your heart with courage, simple faith, and perfect peace. Then she quoted Psalms 31:24 "Be strong and let your heart take courage, all you who hope in the Lord." I am so blessed to have wonderful friends as when I feel like giving up I get an unexpected and so dearly needed uplifting message. Friends that I can share deep fear and doubt that I try to insulate my family from as to try not to worry them.

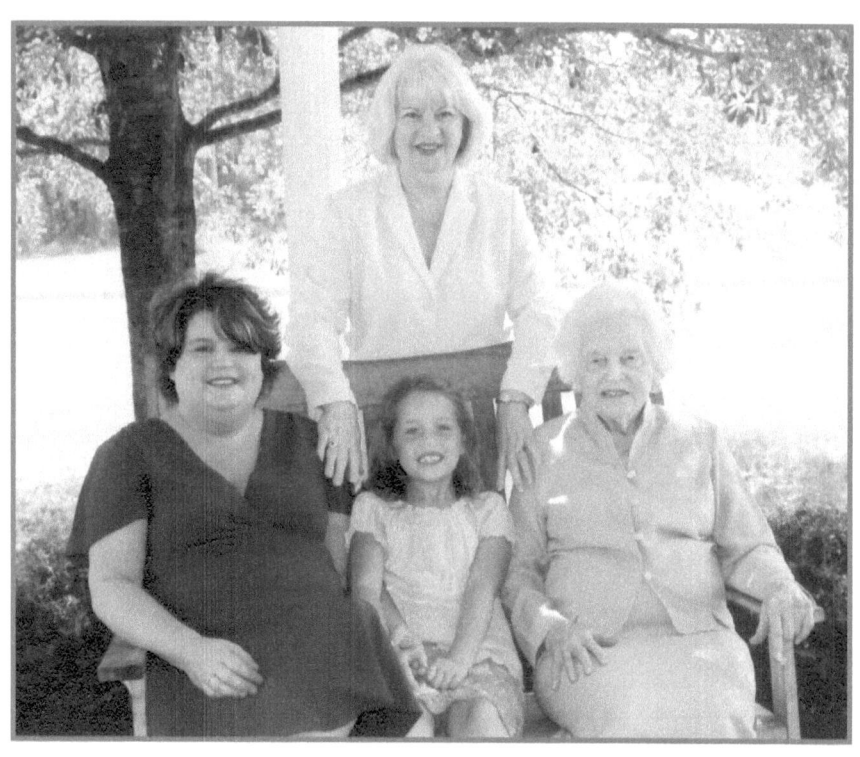

Mother's Day

Chapter 6

Wonderful Mother

I was so happy with my career and the care our staff provided with compassion and love. I was getting better but it had just taken so long. Mother's day was coming and we planned for my mother and brothers to come and also my Aunt Vera. Steve was out of the hospital but still was on continuous oxygen. We had come so close to losing him and he was getting better slowly. I was so excited about the family gathering I could hardly wait to see everyone. I had not been able to visit Steve much when he was in the hospital. I could not get in crowds and had to avoid anyone sick. Mother's Day was also a little sad, my son David would graduate with his Masters in Theology and we had planned for me to travel to LA and go to graduation and spend some time in California. I was not yet strong enough for that trip and would miss his graduation. I was so proud of him. He had worked so hard and was very happy and had been so helpful during this ordeal. Tommy was back in the hospital and I prayed daily he would get his life back and destroy the monsters that plagued him day and night. I hurt so badly for him, he was trying and I knew he would do anything to get better. I still had the feeding tube, but was eating better and should be able to get it out soon. Cancer is so hard on our bodies. We don't know until we feel the fight. I planned to go to church on Sunday and hoped my energy would be better. I did go back to work and was anxious to see everyone. My boss had been wonderful and I had already been out 6 months and he continued my insurance and that was so important. I thank God for such a wonderful boss and enjoyed working for him. I knew I needed to return and get ready for our survey due in September. The staff and residents were happy I was back and made me feel so good. I felt they were good medicine, I was more determined not to let cancer take over my life. I must fight and try to help others that are tired, weak, afraid and in pain from the horrible effects of cancer and the task of just getting through the treatment. I still had moments that I wondered Why? I was a good person; my career was taking care and helping others. Why? Why? Why me?? Then I think why not you, who do you think you are? I will never be proud I got cancer, everyone you love and loves you also hurts, but I will try to be proud of the way I handled it and tried to fight to survive and be able to help others that will have all the fear and doubts I had. God please help me to get better and not become bitter. I will continue to do all I can to get better and stronger. Remember I am not in control.

The June meeting at Amelia Island was a perfect time to get some rest and spend the week with Bob and no chores or phone calls. This was a beautiful location and the beach was so close you could open the doors and hear the ocean. Bob and I had a lot of wonderful memories at Amelia Island. I planned long walks on the beach in the moonlight, good seafood and making love to the sound of the ocean waves. The sounds were so relaxing and seem to say everything is right. You are so blessed by this God that controls the universe. The reality was I could not go down to the beach, my energy was so low I just made it to the walkway and looked at Bob. He said let's go back to the room and sit on the patio. I agreed and we walked very slow back to the entrance and got on the elevator, when the door closed I reached over and hugged Bob. He smiled and said you know the elevator has a camera, don't overdo it. I smiled and tried to hold the tears in. I did not have the energy to walk down to the beach; I would not have the energy to make love. Bob got us a coke and we sat on the patio and watched the sun go down. We had dinner in the room and went to bed Bob held me gently and let me rest. I told him I had planned to make passionate love to him. He said we will when you have more energy. He kissed me and said you owe me, giving me that naughty smile I loved. I secretly prayed and I asked God to give me enough energy to handle love making soon. I had a wonderful husband that loved me and not once complained. He said I want you to get stronger and we know it will take time. Be patient it is going to get better, it is already better you are not hurting and you are not taking medicine for Nausea. Yes, I said but I want to feel normal. I said I do owe you back rubs, baths, meals and many romantic nights. He was teasing me but I owed him so much, I will never forget him rubbing my back and feet, bringing me food and water writing down my schedule and medication times. But, most of all making me feel like a woman when I had lost so much weight. I felt like a small child in bed. I had always had a round, firm booty and he loved my body, Now I had no booty, I told Bob when I get my booty back I know I will be on the mend back to health. He said you will get it back. It would just take time. I did not say anything but I though it should be back already. Then that little voice in my head said Thank you God for healing me. Claim it and believe it don't let doubt in. Please God help me believe and feel better. I miss energy and feeling playful. Reality and coping at work everyone had been so helpful, but my energy was so low I could not do all I wanted. I mostly stayed at my desk. The best part of working in a nursing home is the time you spend with the residents. I loved making rounds and visiting with each resident. Each visit is so special and always a surprise and their appreciation for the attention made me feel like I really was making a difference in their day. I have so many fond memories of my career in Long Term Care. I could write a novel about the lessons they have taught me. I always walked away with a special memory. That will be my next book. When cancer and it's awful weakness is over. Doctor Giraldo had scheduled a MRI for the numbness and pain in my neck and shoulder. The MRI showed degenerative disc in the area I had received radiation C-3-4-5-6-7. Now I had another Doctor. I would follow up with her and see If I could avoid more surgery. It took a month to get an appointment. I have been disappointed in how long you have to wait to get any appointment with a specialist. Dear God I need patience. I decided I needed to stop work. I cannot do all I need to and it is not right to hold on to this wonderful job. My boss had not complained about all the time I had taken, but as a manager I knew it was not right. I called Mr. Charles and explained it to him. He said take a couple of weeks and see if you feel better; you may need a little more time. I agreed and thanked him. After the two weeks I was still very weak and decided to tell Mr. Charles to find someone. I would cover until he found someone. I was so sad, because I loved my job, but I hated not doing it with the passion and energy I needed.

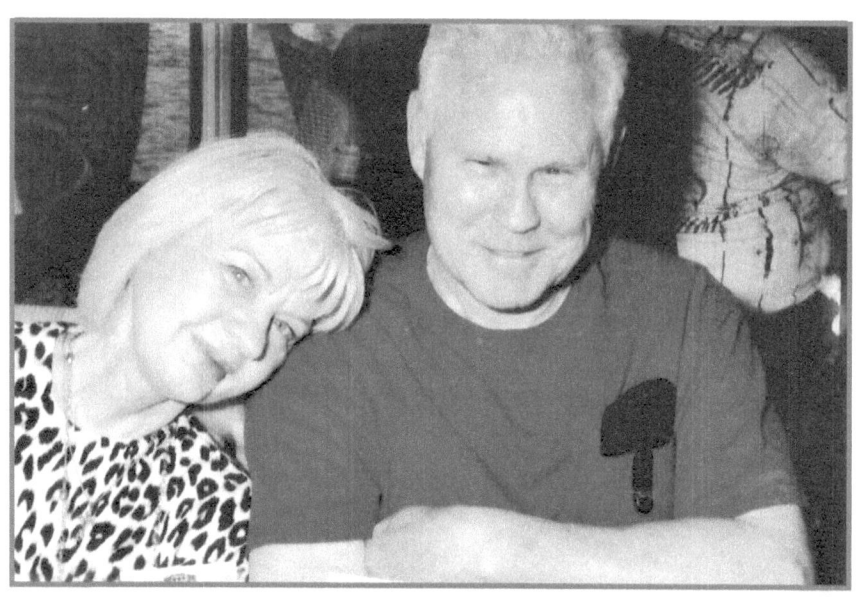

My Rock

Chapter 7

Acceptance

I realize more and more how our health care is in a crisis, how would I continue health Insurance? I knew my diagnosis would keep me unable to obtain insurance, if I let my insurance go. I knew it would be very expensive and not working would put a strain on our budget, Bob said 'Do not worry, we will be able to do it. Remember I made the vow through sickness and in health" If I could qualify for disability it would still be 2 years before I would be covered on Medicare. What should I do I had worked 30 years in health care and had saved for retirement, but one hospitalization with extensive treatment could put us in poverty and deeply in debt. We all plan to work until we have Medicare or retirement insurance. We don't plan cancer, pain, and disability. I will continue to fight this cancer and trust that I will get well and feel healthy again. I read a poem that stated what cancer can't take away love, faith and hope. Tomorrow I will have the PET scan. This should be the last chapter for my survival book. That will tell that I have no cancer left, that is our prayers and hopes we have not talked out loud about what if, but I think about it. I am no longer working and have felt better the last week. I need to take care of some other health problems but can't think beyond tomorrow now. We can plan to celebrate no cancer and then work on my neck and female problems. I want to look in the eyes of my children and say we beat this awful cancer and lay in Bob's arms and not wonder what will happen next. God I have tried to have total faith and believe I will overcome this horrible disease and be an example for others that face the battle with such a demon as cancer. I feel close to God but still have fear, I am so confused, others seem not to ever doubt and fear. God forgive me for doubting and help me to do your wonderful will. God help Tommy he is hurting so badly, we don't understand but you already know the answer for him. Tomorrow will bring hope and survival. I just have to believe. The Pet Scan showed some uptake in the tongue, That concerns me but Doctor Gourin said not to worry it was probably form the radiation. I still have swelling and tenderness from the radiation. We will have to repeat the PET scan in 3 or 4 months I will see Doctor Gourin again in 6 weeks. Nothing is simple in Cancer Care. I will continue to hope and pray. Michelle, a friend of my son, David, called stated she would continue the healing touch by remote. This is a process of healing touch and relaxation; I will do all things possible to beat this cancer. I saw Doctor Christine and she would try to give me some relief of the severe stiffness in my neck by cutting the paroxysmal band. This was scheduled for October 26th at MCG. The surgery went well and I recovered quickly. The surgery did help some, and I was resting much better at night. I would have to continue follow up and have my mouth and neck checked every 2 months for another year. We are celebrating every month with a grateful heart that we were able to fight this horrible disease of cancer. I do know that I will always fear the return but will rremember the words posted in the lobby of the Oncologist that states.

Cancer cannot take away hope, love, joy, family, and salvation. Yes, it is hard and don't believe for a moment you want have a lot of fear. But you still have hope when all else fails. Your life is precious, and enjoy where you are every day.

Cancer Cannot:

Cripple Love

Shatter Hope

Corrode Faith

Destroy Peace

Kill Friendships

Suppress Memories

Silence Courage

Invade the Soul

Steal Eternal Life

Conquer the Spirit

I needed more surgery. Doctor Christine had left MCG, and accepted a position at John Hopkins, I was glad for her career, but could not imagine not seeing her. She had been so reassuring when times were the hardest. She left Doctor Jackson in charge of my care and sure enough she was also wonderful. The stiffness and hardness became very difficult to deal with and I started dropping everything I picked up. My primary physician referred me to a neurologist. Doctor Ellen scheduled surgery. I would have 3 disc removed and a cage placed around Them to stabilize my spine. A plastic surgeon would also transfer some tissue to help the stiffness in my neck. After the surgery I wore a cervical collar 6 weeks and also the PET Scan was repeated and was now completely normal. We will celebrate after

I recover from the surgery. The radiation did a lot of damage but the cancer is gone. In May 2008 I published a children's book entitled "Mema Has Cancer" to show how our precious grandchildren dealt with me not being able to play as before. We had to change a lot of things in our life and now we are so thankful that soon we can start a new chapter and say now I am cancer free and will always celebrate each new day. Follow up with Doctor Jackson on June 3rd, I look forward to that visit. She was there for the neck resection and knows the entire history. She will tell me how often we will have to do the Pet Scans.

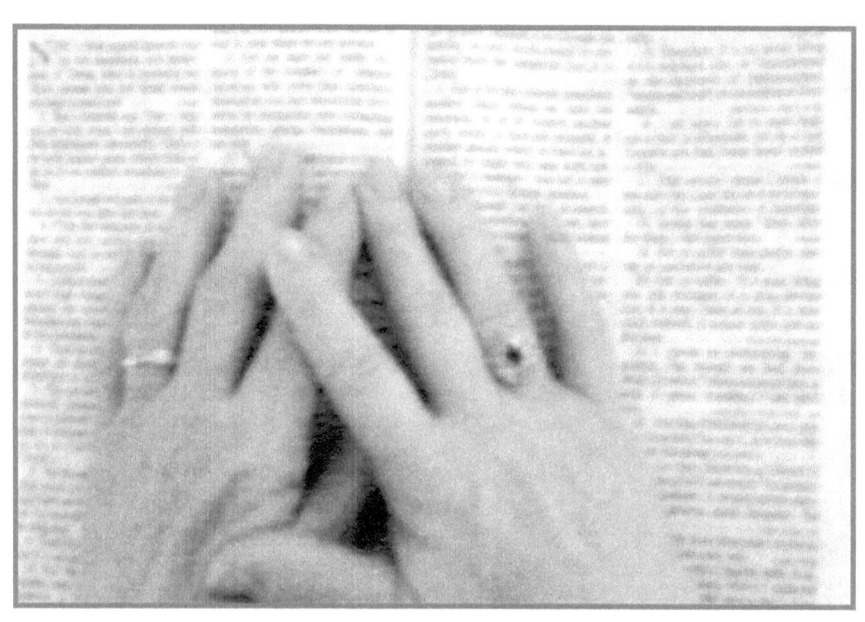

I will Love my Hands

Chapter 8

Reality

Life is about living. I want to be so mindful of how quickly your life can be turned upside down and do everything possible to stay happy and healthy. Thinking about all the hard lessons learned, dealing with divorce, family crisis, illnesses makes me realize how soon our world can be turned upside down. We can learn so much from our darkest times. When I look into my first born eyes, I see the pain that his challenges have caused him and wonder why. When he told me about his lifestyle, I feared his acceptance in the work place, in the church, in our family or just walking down the street. I have been blessed to have two sons. My youngest son is a minister that has touched so many lives with love, compassion, and empathy. The world is a better place because he is here. My daughter is a wonderful mother to my grandchildren. I know we all will have times when we question Why, Why?? Then think and say, Why not??. You can and will learn so much from your hardest times. Don't they say when you are in the valley you remember how wonderful the mountain was. June 1st was a beautiful clear day and we were going to church. We walked in and went to the row we always sat. I was happy to see our church family, they had fixed food and delivered each time I had surgery. We were so blessed to have this church family. Brother Brown welcomed the congregation and gave the Scripture, 2 Corinthians Chapter 11. I turned to the scripture and realized how dependent my right hand had become. His sermon was very well prepared and then it was time for communion. I had not had communion in a long time and I felt thankful to be there. The prayer was said and the deacons passed the silver tray with the Communion bread. Brother James put the tray in front of me and my finger and thumb would not work together I tried my left hand and after three tries I picked up the bread that represented the body of Christ that suffered and died that we have an abundant life. I was now doing all I could not to burst out in tears. I would not look up. I felt Bobs hand on my shoulder but I could not look up. I knew I could not hold back the sobs if I looked at him. Another prayer was said and I put the bread in my mouth. I knew it was time for the communion wine to be served and I said God please help me to partake and not spill your blood. When the silver tray was passed Bob held it very close for me. I picked it up and waited for the prayer. Brother Brown said drink in remembrance of our Lord and Savior. I swallowed the wine and again said God please help me. I placed my cup in the pew holder and realized Bob did not take communion. He was so concerned about me and had his doubt in himself and his relationship with God. He had been my rock and if anyone was ever worthy to partake of communion, it was Bob. I wanted to tell him that as we walked to the car, but he looked at me and said are you all right. I burst into uncontrollable tears and said I could hardly pick up the communion bread. He said but you did and you are here and you are so much better. I said I know and I feel so bad that I am complaining but all the emotions are so fresh again. He said you have been through so much, it is OK to cry. He was so compassionate I was glad we were almost home. He said we will have a sandwich for lunch, then take a nap. I walked into the kitchen, Bob was making us a glass of tea, the phone rang, Bob answered and it was Amanda. He gave me the phone and Amanda told me that Hannah would be going to the sitter on Monday. I said OK, and she said what is wrong? I did not want her to know how upset I was, but I told her about Communion and she said but you are so much better. I know I should be so thankful for my survival that I would not moan over the loss of control in my hands. I was mourning now, because I loved my life and I missed all the things I took for granted before. I was having a pity party, and missing the simple things like writing, putting on mascara, signing my name, driving, cutting my toe nails, singing and being in control of my hands. June 4th I saw Doctor Jackson; she did a scope and said everything looked good. She will see me again in 8 weeks. My therapist told me I was doing well, but you need to be patient. You want to be perfect and that may not happen. Damaged nerves heal slowly and may never be the way they were before the damage. She smiled at me and said, I am so proud of your hard work, but it may take months; but keep working on the hard things and it will get easier. My granddaughter said Mema just slow down and learn to print, that will be easy. The wisdom in the eyes of a child, I will practice I told her. Now, Mema let's go to McDonald's. I called Amanda to pick us up and take Hannah to McDonald's. Life can be simple when we listen to our grandchildren.

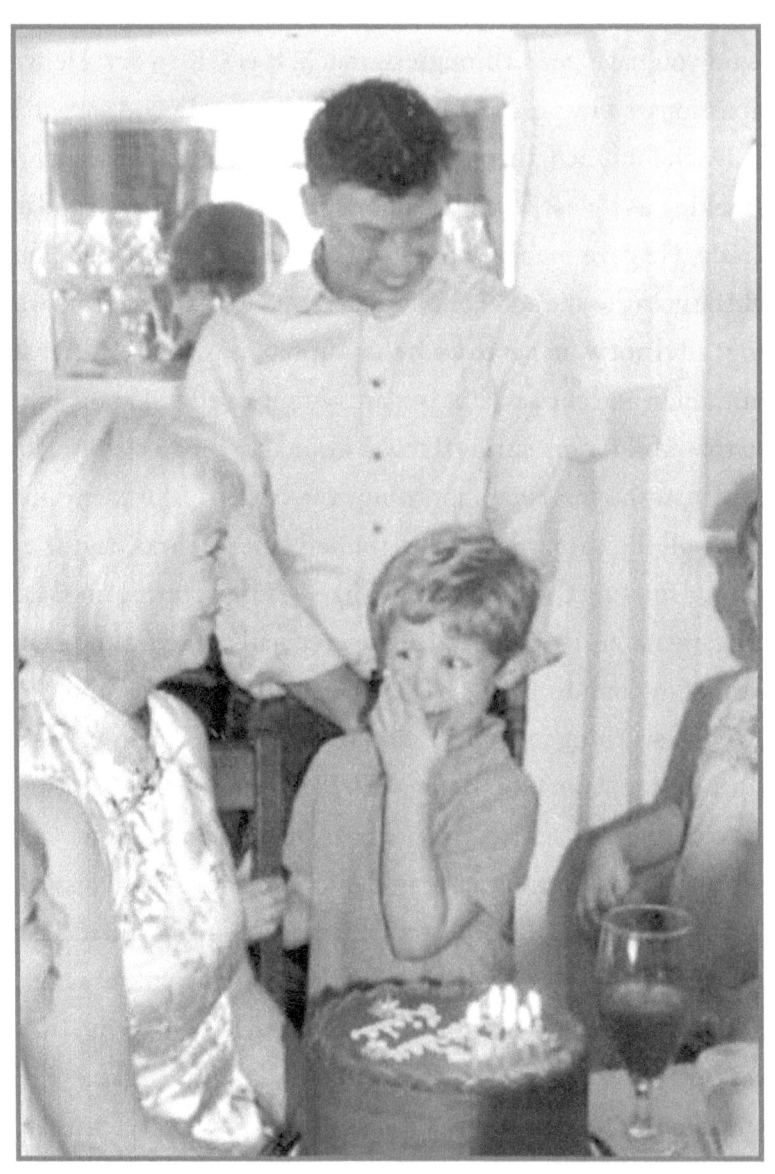

You are my Sunshine

Chapter 9

Cheers to Another Birthday

I will plan a trip to California for David's birthday; this will be the time we send in the children's book "Mema Has Cancer" to be published. I am so excited about the children's book that was inspired by my granddaughter Hannah. I have been blessed and with time I will gain more control in my hand, but I will never take the simple things in life for granted again. Dear God please help me brush my teeth tonight. I will wake up and need you again tomorrow. Since Doctor Christine left and went to John Hopkins I have been seeing Doctor Jackson every two months to make sure no reoccurrence of the cancer. In September my children gave me a wonderful 60th birthday party. Family, friends and fellow workers came to celebrate. Friends from church and childhood made the day so full of love. This will be a wonderful memory forever. My granddaughters sang You Are my

Sunshine and added the words please do not take my Mema away. I could not hold back the tears of joy and the room was full of love. I had been concerned it seemed that I was dropping almost everything. I saw a neurologist and he sent me for another MRI. This showed some suspicious glands. This meant more surgery. I went in on December 22nd and the biopsy was negative. "Thank you God!" I said over and over again. Now we would try to find out what was wrong with my hands. My son David wrote me a beautiful letter. He said mom I want you to read this every morning. Put it where you will remember to read it each morning I want nothing more for you than to be able to move to the next stage of your recovery. I love you.

My hands are unable to do what they once did. No matter how much I expect from them, they will not do what they cannot do. Today I will be honest with myself, heart, mind and body as I accept that my hands are no longer under my control. I will begin to love my hands that have always been there for me. I will start to understand the limits they are now facing. They are the victims of the war that was fault and won. It was not their choice. I do not blame them. I will watch them daily I will accept them as they are. Loving them more today than yesterday and expecting less from them today than yesterday. Today I will love my disabled hands. I will love my handicap hands. I will love my special-needs hands. I will love my slow hands. I will love my challenged hands. I will love my diminished hands. I will love my crippled hands. I will love my hands. When the right one drops and hurts, I will kiss it gently with love. When the Left one refuses to hold its own, and numbly aches, I will kiss it gently with love. They are mine. Today I will love my hands.

This has made my days brighter. Thank you David for such inspiring words as you always know what to say and when to say it. I look forward to a big hug and holding your hand. I will see my new doctor this week. He is going to try to inject Botox into my hands. Hopefully this will give me some better control and use. Each day I thank God that I can do what I do, but I also want so much more. I want to shop, go to a beauty shop, play with the grand kids, color and paint. I have not been able to take care of my plants and have a garden for three years. I feel selfish, but long to be normal. Each visit to the doctor I see so many much worse than me and I remember I have no right to question, why this happened to me. I will continue to pray and believe I will survive.

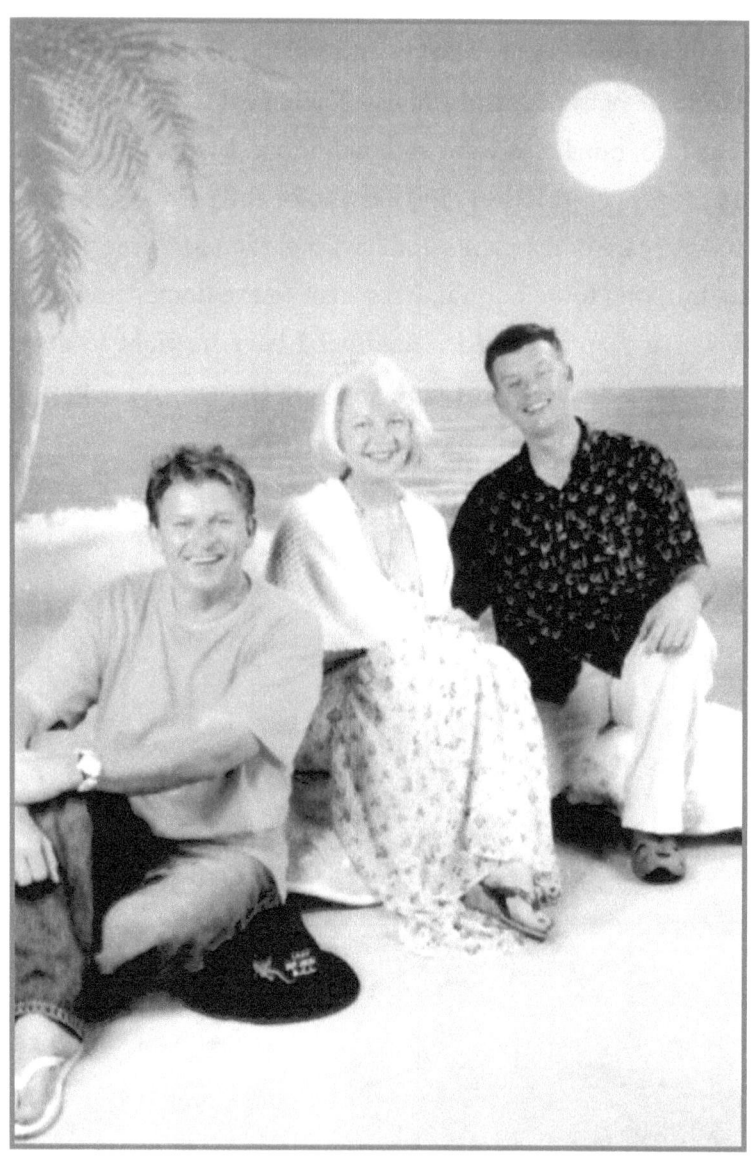

Gma we're here

Chapter 10

Graduation

octor Robertson graduated me. That was his words, as he looked smiling at me. He saw the puzzled look on my face, and said you are 4 years clean and I think you have beat this cancer. He said but call me if you ever need me. I said thanks so much for everything, you have been wonderful. I sat there not thinking for a long minute. Thank you God, I want to tell MaMa her prayers were answered, she always believed I would be healed. But, Mom died in hospice June 20, 2010. She had fallen in April, suffered a fracture in cervical spine. She hated the fact of being dependent and needing more assistance. We laid in her queen size bed and had wonderful talks while she stayed in the personal care home. She was scheduled for follow up x-ray and the neurologist said the fracture was healing. I felt relief that soon she would get out of the neck brace. She was scheduled for a bone scan the following Monday. Mom had had her house up for sale, for several months and received the call it was sold. She had mixed emotions, she knew she would not be able to move back into her home, but wanted to see the pears, figs, and grapes come in another season. We had so many wonderful memories of the home place where she and Dad had loved so much. I cried when I thought of all she had given up. We talked about the last night we had stayed, she reminded me she had said then this is too much on me getting around in the house. She said I hope it sells soon and the family that lives here will take care of it. I agreed and just like that, she had a buyer. Her prayers were answered. Her lawyer and his wife visited her in the personal care home. She enjoyed their visit, they had been friends over 50 years, and he knew every detail of her business. She laughed as they shared old stories. When I came in the room he said he would handle the closing and the visit was great and he knew mom was competent to make her own decisions. He smiled and told her, you are sharp, you remember better than me. Mom loved that, she took pride in staying sharp. So the week before the bone scan she had sold her house and talked with her lawyer to make sure all her affairs were in order. I did not know she had also talked with the funeral director, to make sure he had all her request written out. Saturday morning we moved all the things out of the house to be stored until we knew what to do with everything. When I got home Mom called and said she needed me she was in terrible pain. I grabbed my purse and left. I was just 10 minutes away. I knew she was in a lot of pain because she was not a complainer. As soon as I got to the room she could not move without severe pain in her hip. I called home health and her Doctor. Home Health Nurse, Janie came right out, called the Doctor got orders for pain medication and a catheter, she would not have to get up. They decided she was already scheduled for scan on Monday and if the pain medication worked, it would be best to wait for the bone scan. She would be carried by ambulance to the hospital Monday morning and we would know what the treatment plan would be. I was not prepared for the scan results. Doctor Aaron came in after the scan and said, Mom had multiple fractures and severe deterioration of bones. He recommended inpatient hospice and comfort measures. Mom asked when. He said I will talk with the team and make sure we have done all we need to do. He patted her hand and said you let us know if you need anything, she said thank you. I could not believe all this was happening so fast. I called my brothers, then I called my kids, David was in California, I knew he would want to come. The room became so busy. I looked at Mom, she looked good, but they said hospice. That week is a blur. Friday she was transferred to hospice house and was made pain free and comfortable.. I just did not know the end was so near. She was excited when David came in and they talked until late Saturday night, my brother and his wife were spending the night. I kissed Mom on the forehead and said goodnight. Sunday morning Tommy and David went in to see Mom and Tommy said G-Ma we are here, David said let her rest and she took her last breath. The phone rang I thought it was the girls calling to wish Bob happy Father's Day, one word from Bob and I knew something was so wrong. He said we will be there soon as possible. I still feel shocked as to how fast it happened. We just never know. I was blessed to be raised by wonderful parents and I had a wonderful Christian Mother for 89 years, I miss her daily and hope I will be so strong when I am on my last day.

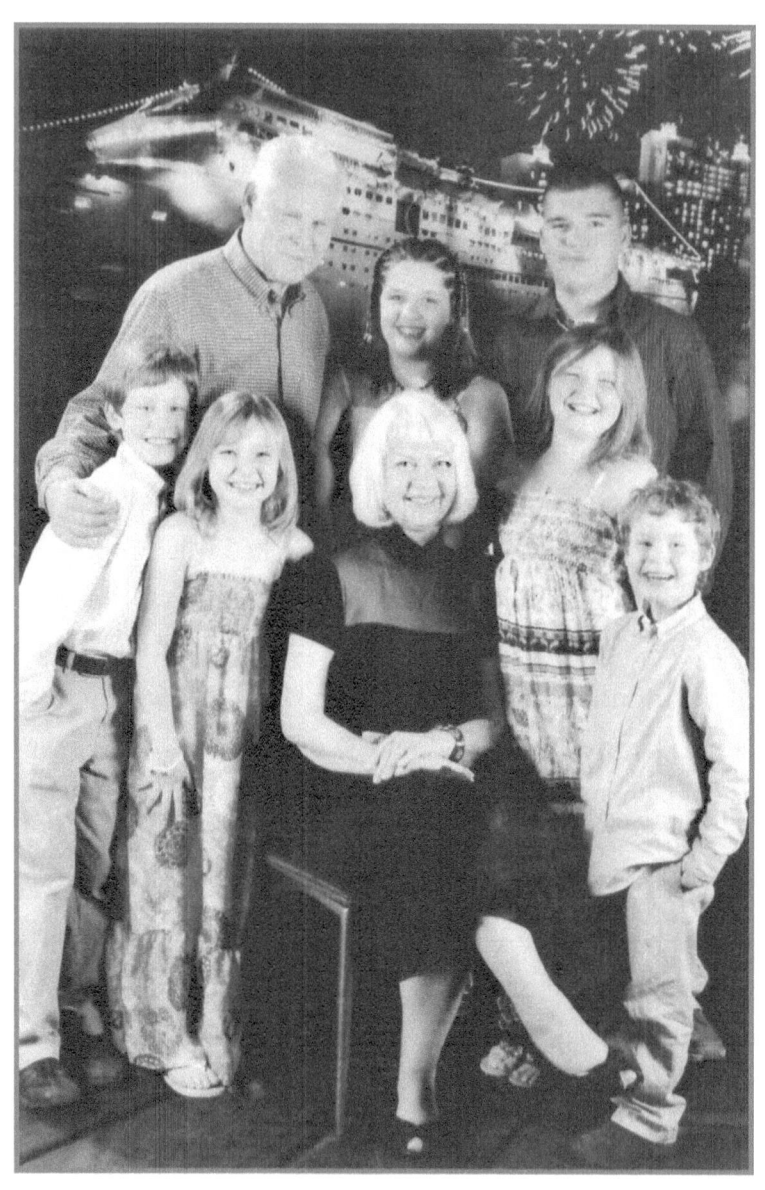

Lullaby of Hope

Chapter 11

Elation

We did do a book signing for "Me Ma Has Cancer" this book will help children understand the struggles of family members going through cancer treatment. So I can say something good did come from this horrible disease. Cancer has changed my life. Cancer has changed the life of my family. Today my son Tommy is vigilant in maintaining a healthy lifestyle. How many mothers can say that her son whom has dealt with so many personal trials would recently post this message to me on Facebook: Mama I love you and thank God for you every day. I am so blessed to have your uncompromising love and support. I may question a lot of things in my life but one truth is always the same. I am loved and so thankful for having been looked upon by my Angels to have you as my Mother. My daughter Amanda is taking better care of herself and has achieved her dream of a college degree in

Criminal Justice fulfilling her passion and making a difference. My son David is helping others deal with grief and upset in accepting that bad things do happen, but we can fight every day to survive and share our hope, doubt, and fears. His play entitled Caught ran for 9 months in Los Angeles at the Zephyr theatre and is now scheduled for a reading in New York City with the dream and potential of Broadway. I will work hard to regain my strength to do the things I love and look forward to attending his opening night on Broadway. I love my life with Bob and pray I will soon be the active woman he married. He has been there through the darkest days and never complained. I only hope I will soon give him all I have promised. I owe him big. Enjoy every moment of your life. Refuse to be discouraged. Refuse to give up. Love Your Life!!! I want to participate in relay for life this year. My emotions have been so raw that I could not even speak about it last year. I hope this year I will be an active part in the encouragement of other cancer patients. I did not walk in the relay for life. I made a contribution, but had just heard my niece Kelly had a report that her cancer had spread, I was afraid again of this reminder you are never the same. I know I am so blessed and have passed the five year mark. I will enjoy every moment and try not to moan with all the side effects. Tommy wrapped it all up for me, when he said, after one day during my pity party. Mom you are alive, we have you. He is right, but more important, I HAVE THEM. THANK YOU FOR A SECOND CHANCE.

www.ingramcontent.com/pod-product-compliance
Lightning Source LLC
Chambersburg PA
CBHW021303280526
45784CB00005B/2499